The Drinker's Manifesto © 2019 by Better Drinking Culture

Contact the publisher:
Better Drinking Culture, PBC
betterdrinkingculture.org | hello@betterdrinkingculture.org

ISBN-13: 978-1-7325059-0-2
ISBN-10: 1-7325059-0-X

Printed in the United States of America
Ingram Printing & Distribution, 2019

Written by Jason Ley | jasonley.com | @jasonley
Direction by Camden Brieden
Layout by Svannah Nguyen and Joshua Best
Administrative assistance by Katherine Ley
Edited by Steven Michael Holmes

To the OG BDC Tribe:
Camden, Selina, TJ, Lindsay, Michael, Rachel, AB, Lauren, Wes, Taylor, Amy, Jim, Madison, Alex, Jimmy, Kris, Brett, Mike, Jeff, Jon, Douglas, Amie, Dave, MacKenzie, Dina, Nate, Eric, Anne, Rachel, Kevin, Karen, Dick, Motu, Andy, Ryan, April, Joe, Lisa, Robb, Mark, Dixie, Kylee, Sam, Max, and everyone else who supported the BDC in our early days. Thank you!

First Edition

BETTER
DRINKING
CULTURE

THE DRINKER'S
MANIFESTO

CHEERS TO A BETTER DRINKING CULTURE

To our friends who founded the movement,
for the tribe who now owns it.

CONTENTS

FOREWORD

was drunk the first time I learned about Better Drinking Culture. Technically, I was sober *at first*. It was June 11, 2015, in Grand Rapids, Michigan. A trusted friend and respected mentor invited me to a new beer-and-food pairing event that he conceptualized with the polite request for my feedback about what I thought worked and what didn't. That event just happened to be the first time BDC formally organized in public since quietly launching a few months earlier.

When I walked in, the first thing I noticed was that at every brewery's station there was someone pouring beer who was wearing a different colored T-shirt that read BETTER DRINKING CULTURE. The name alone piqued my interest. I was intrigued.

I spent the next couple hours immersing myself in the experience so that I could make good on my promise to advise with recommendations. In the meantime, I exhausted all of my comped drink tickets. On my way out, now intoxicated, I felt compelled to stop by the BDC merch table. I can't remember who I talked to— you can probably guess why, but I asked the guy to tell me about Better Drinking Culture. His response— BDC's mission—cut straight through my buzzed-up, fuzzy state. The first thing out of my mouth: "Where were you when I was in college?"

I graduated from Michigan State University in 2001 with a bachelor's degree in English and a minor in binge drinking. I have the literal scars to show that I put too much time into "studying" for the latter. The day after I walked across the stage to accept my diploma, I spent the afternoon in the emergency room having my right hand stitched back together because I smashed a half-gallon of liquor while wasted at my own graduation party.

Just about every regret or moment of shame I have that has made it too painful to look myself in the mirror was conceived at the bottom of a bottle that I had no business emptying. I have lost my balance and stumbled to the edge countless times, somehow barely dodging my own rock-bottom.

Fast-forward to the fall of 2016. I got an unsolicited

email from BDC's co-founder, Camden Brieden, who found me through a TV show I created about the craft beer scene. He introduced himself, and wrote, "I would love to connect to learn more about the projects you're working on, and share some ideas and a vision I have that could lead to some shared opportunities." I still can't say with certainty who I talked to from BDC the year prior—it very well could've been, and probably was, Cam. What are the chances?

I took Cam up on his offer, and we met for lunch. He ordered a water, and I ordered a beer. We clicked. So much in fact that he invited me out to lunch again three weeks later. I didn't realize in that moment that I was walking into a final job interview. Toward the end of our meal, he casually asked me about what my drinking was like in college. While recounting one of the many stories I wish I could take back and rewrite, I started tearing up from pulling the scab off an old, painful wound. He sat there across from me as I was trying to regain my composure. He nodded with compassion as if he understood what I was saying better than I did. With as much sensitivity as one person could embody, Cam gently asked, "Would you like to take over leading BDC?"

I wrote *The Drinker's Manifesto* from the point of view of Better Drinking Culture. However, I wrote it *to* who I was in college, to everyone I've drank too much with, and to the current generation of drinkers and college students with the hope that they would feel empowered to pass down a drinking culture for future generations *better* than the one that was left for us. Better than the way it was left for my friends and me. And better than the way I almost left it for you.

When Cam asked me if I'd consider writing the *Foreword*, which wasn't part of our original plan because it would oddly be for the same book I also just wrote, I gave him the same answer I did when he trusted me to run BDC. I couldn't *not* do it.

I'm human, and still make mistakes, but I care and I try. Believing in a better drinking culture and walking it out are not synonymous with perfection, but with love, intent, and grace. We're not in this alone.

I sincerely hope that this book does for you the same thing it could've done for me.

Now, go be awesome.

Jason Ley, CEO
Better Drinking Culture

PREFACE

ello. We're Better Drinking Culture. You can call us BDC. *The Drinker's Manifesto* is a culmination of our desires to build a better drinking culture for ourselves and our friends. Our hope is that— if we develop a greater respect for what we drink, we can deepen the respect for our relationship with alcohol.

We wrote this book because we were sick and tired of waking up feeling like crap and regretting what we did the night before—if we even remembered it. Our lives can either be joyfully enhanced or completely obliterated when we drink. Our culture has historically glorified the over-consumption of alcohol. More

> **"**
> We wrote this book because we were sick and tired of waking up feeling like crap.

than just encouraging us to drink, our culture *expects* us to—*a lot*.

This widespread, normalized phenomenon has contributed to influencing people to misuse alcohol because drinking is promoted as cool, fun, and harmless. These messages can be found embedded almost anywhere alcohol is present—some of which are more subtle than others, while many are blatant and shameless. Too many of us have learned the hard way after putting ourselves or someone else in harm's way. When we come to the sobered-up realization that getting wasted leads to an onslaught of negative consequences, we find out that the path to social acceptance that our culture is selling us has a false bottom.

> **"**
> Yet, a better way of drinking is rarely, if ever, promoted with the same enthusiasm.

Yet, a better way of drinking is rarely, if ever, promoted with the same enthusiasm.

So, we decided to do something about it. We ignited a movement to set the example for the next generation. We're intent on leaving this place better than how we found it. We wanted better for ourselves, and we want better for you.

Before we go any further, we want to tell you how

Better Drinking Culture got here. Camden Brieden, BDC's co-founder, has a story. It just so happens to be the prelude to BDC.

Back in high school, a classmate once told me, "You're going to look back at your life and wish you partied harder." We were at a typical house party: no parents and tons of cheap alcohol. And, like every other party I had been to, I was the only one not drinking.

Although most of the people I knew in school drank whenever they had a chance, I was really fortunate that my friends and I shared a mutual respect for each other, including our decisions to drink or not drink. My choice to not drink was heavily influenced by my family, specifically my mother who, at that time, was struggling with her relationship with alcohol.

> **❝**
> What I quickly learned was that everyone had a story.

Growing up in a family negatively impacted by alcohol was not easy. Sharing this openly with my friends? Much harder. But, I cared deeply about my mom and learned as much as I could about the science of addiction. Once I fully understood that addiction was not a character flaw or weakness, but rather a complex condition of the brain, I was better equipped to share my story with my friends. What I quickly learned was that everyone had a story about how drinking too much had negatively impacted their life or the life of someone they knew. Stories of

17

regret, lost memories, weekends wasted, relationships ruined. The list almost doesn't have an end. And most of them on the spectrum of "I cannot believe I did that last night" are often hidden in plain sight.

We discovered a common thread through sharing these stories: **Nearly every negative consequence related to alcohol was the result of drinking too much.** *It wasn't alcohol alone. It was drinking too much of it. And then came the big idea! If we choose to drink better, all of these negative experiences would never happen in the first place.*

> **"**
> Nearly every negative consequence related to alcohol was the result of drinking too much.

So, I invited the same group of friends who shared their stories with me back into the conversation. We sat down together over drinks (some with alcohol, some without) and drafted a manifesto of what a "better drinking culture" looks like. We built a simple website, shared our stories on it, printed some shirts, and planted a flag firmly in the ground for what we believed to be a better way. It didn't take long before people from all corners of the globe started sharing their stories with us, repping BDC shirts, and spreading the love with their friends. It was honest, authentic, simple, and sincere.

Looking back today at my life, I don't regret not partying "harder." I had an absolute blast in high school and college.

> **"**
> I don't regret not partying 'harder.'

I just did it without alcohol. Even to this day, I still haven't had a drop. Not one. I'm proud of my choice. Yours may be different than mine, and that's okay. BDC was founded by drinkers and non-drinkers—by the very people who choose to consume alcohol as well as those who equally choose not to. BDC is not a campaign, it's a lifestyle.

> "
> We're a movement of people who believe in something better, and everyone's invited.

It's not a product of the industry or a university. We're a movement of people who believe in something better, and everyone's invited.

We *all* have a story. If it's not about us, it's likely about someone we know, someone we love, or someone we miss. And, all of our stories still share that singular underlying theme: *Nearly every negative consequence associated with alcohol is the result of drinking too much.* If we can educate and empower people to drink better and live healthier we'll be able to look back on our lives and tell the story of a life that we not only remember fondly, but one that we're proud of living.

BDC's mission is to shift our culture's relationship with alcohol in a healthier and more positive direction—encouraging a lifestyle free from pain, harm, and regret. Because hangovers suck.

INTRODUCTION

The purpose of *The Drinker's Manifesto* is to educate, empower, and equip anyone who decides to drink to do so better, and to encourage others to do the same.

To be clear, BDC is not anti-alcohol. As a matter of fact, many of us love a good drink and the camaraderie that comes with sharing a cold one with our friends. Nor is this book an endorsement to start drinking. If you're already there we'll never try to entice you with the pressure of, "C'mon, just one more!" Instead, we want you to have the wherewithal to make that decision for yourself.

We're here to support you on your journey, even if you stumble along the way. If this was a trust fall, we'd catch you. You don't have to sign an oath in blood to live a healthier lifestyle. Don't let a misconception that you have to be mistake-free in your relationship with alcohol weigh you down. BDC doesn't "kick you out" if you have a rough night with the bottle. You don't have to carry the weight of yesterday's baggage. We'll never judge or shame you. Regardless of where you are currently and how much you (may or may not) drink, today is a new opportunity.

Better Drinking Culture is unique in that we are both drinkers and non-drinkers. You don't have to drink to believe in BDC. We're an anomaly like that, and we like it that way. We owe no allegiances except to ourselves. We're free agents of our own accord.

If you were to pull back the curtain on BDC, you won't find a major corporation pulling the strings. We're not a government agency or a political party funded by lobbyists with a hidden agenda. We're not a coalition that's trying to convince you that we're cool or hip. We're not your parents. We may not even be friends yet, but we are people who care.

BDC is reestablishing the rules of engagement for what it means to drink or to be a "drinker." We're setting the bar higher than it's been held for how we should respect ourselves, what we drink, and for a culture that wants to curate better drinkers. For us, drinking better means drinking mindfully—a conscious approach to consuming. You've heard the saying, "All good things in moderation." We can get behind that. Essentially, we believe people should drink within their own personal limits.

> **"**
> Drinking better means drinking mindfully.

The Drinker's Manifesto is organized into three main parts: *Better, Drinking,* and *Culture. Better* lays the foundation for the reasons we choose to drink better, and how doing so can positively affect our health, relationships, and community. *Drinking* outlines practical ways to be mindful about yourself, what you're consuming, and the environment around you while you're drinking. *Culture* is where the shift happens. The decision to be a leader among your peers—a conduit for social impact and a voice for long-term change—is yours.

> **"**
> We believe people should drink within their own personal limits.

As you read this book, take into consideration the following. We're not making assumptions about where you've been in your relationship with alcohol, accusations about where you currently may be, nor criticisms for somewhere you're not. There may be times throughout this book when you roll your eyes at us. We know cynicism is a result of being influenced by skewed, unrealistic social norms. The pressure to do what's cool often overrides being compelled to do what's right.

Lastly, to be fair, this book is not intended for those with a serious drinking problem or a dependency on alcohol. For anyone who may be struggling with an addiction to alcohol or chronically misusing

> **"**
> The pressure to do what's cool often overrides being compelled to do what's right.

it, abstinence may be the only appropriate solution. If that's the case, we encourage you to seek professional help. Instead, *The Drinker's Manifesto* was written for an audience who is either curious about entertaining a lifestyle that includes alcohol or transitioning to adopt one that includes a more mindful approach.

drink bet·ter \\'driŋk 'be-tər\ *v* **1 a** : to drink mindfully (i.e., originating from a healthy state of mind, with clarity, and maintaining present-moment self-awareness) **b** : to drink in moderation (i.e., within one's own personal limits, not in excess or to the point of a loss of self-control)

#BECAUSEHANGOVERS**SUCK**

PART 1

BETTER
DRINKING
CULTURE

We believe in better. A standard of *better* transcends drinking. It encompasses a holistically healthier (way of) life for both our mind and body and those around us. The obvious symptoms of drinking too much not only have the ability to subdue us for up to a day or more, but the subtle, biological effects may have a much more significant impact over time. Because our immune system and central nervous system operate in close communication, flooding our bodies with an abundance of alcohol challenges both to work harder than they should. Striving to live healthier naturally combats this. Thinking we can simply brush off feeling miserable the morning after by chalking it up to being hungover is shortchanging our potential to live a healthier life.

> **"**
> Being hungover is shortchanging our potential to live a healthier life.

1 BETTER HEALTH

Despite waking up with an aching reminder of missed opportunities from last night, we rarely weigh the pros and cons of drinking too much until it's too late.

HANGOVERS

If you've never had one, consider yourself one of the lucky few. They suck. BDC's first iconic tagline, "Because Hangovers Suck," gets the reaction it does (usually an uncomfortable laugh or silent nod in agreement) because those who've had one know. If you haven't, trust us—it's not worth the initiation, despite our culture's propensity to position it as an expected rite of passage.

> **"**
> Commiserating over hangovers together is a bizarre shared cultural bond.

The warped team spirit between friends commiserating over hangovers together is a bizarre shared cultural bond that more proves misery loves company. Yet, we gauge the amount of fun we had by how awful we feel the next morning. If you suffered the same toilet-hugging effects from engaging in practically any other activity that did as much damage to your body as drinking too much, would you expect to be patted on the back for it? No, you'd be smart enough to not engage in the first place. Would it be appropriate for you to applaud someone else? It's backwards bragging rights. This attempt at social posturing looks more like a lazy slouch.

MORNINGS ARE BETTER WITHOUT HANGOVERS

Immediate gratification can be rather enticing, but check the disclaimer first. Our nearsighted desires almost always come with a debt we'll be on the hook to pay for later. It looks like this...

You wake up, do a double-take to figure out whose bed you're in, and are disgusted by your own morning

> **"**
> We rarely weigh the pros and cons of drinking too much until it's too late.

breath. Your body is noticeably exhausted and dehydrated, and you'd kill for a glass of cold water. Your friends are barely pulling themselves together enough to go grab some food, but the thought of eating right now is enough to make you want to puke. Your guts feel like they're being pushed through a meat grinder. Whatever happens next is going down in the bathroom. Or coming up, if you know what we mean. You feel generally slow, something's off. Your mind doesn't seem to be firing on all cylinders, and

> **"**
> The only real "cure" for a hangover is not getting one in the first place.

you're oddly a little uncoordinated. You just lost your balance and awkwardly stumbled into the door frame trying to leave the room, didn't you? You, my friend, have a hangover—a throbbing, nauseous reminder that you overdid it last night. It's our body telling us, "Not cool."

Headaches, vomiting, and the shakes are the tip of the iceberg. If you're looking for a silver bullet, don't waste your time. You can stop Googling "how to cure a hangover" right now. We know, you've seen the ads promoting magic pills and recovery drinks. Save your money. Spoiler alert! The only real "cure" for a hangover is the only one that won't cost you a dime: not getting one in the first place. Kind of anticlimactic, huh?

There have been numerous studies and research on hangover prevention and cures. Dr. Joris Verster, at Utrecht University, on behalf of the Alcohol Hangover Research Group, an international expert group composed of active researchers in the field of alcohol hangovers (seriously, we can't make this stuff up), concludes that "the only practical way to avoid a hangover is to drink less alcohol."[1]

Don't get us wrong, Sunday Funday is a thing for a reason, but piling more alcohol on top of the amount that your body already hasn't been able to filter out will only extend your hangover. We're all about hanging out on a patio for eats and drinks during a gorgeous afternoon, but be careful thinking that bottomless mimosas at your favorite brunch spot or a Bloody Mary garnished with a slider, chicken wing, and an old sneaker wrapped in bacon are going to do the trick. Sure, you'll catch a buzz. A little hair of the dog may make you feel "better" for an hour or two, but you won't be able to outrun the crash by trying to prolong the inevitable.

Okay, so what gives? Are there any hangover hacks?! You're not going to like this, but we've got to burst the bubble on a few of the most popular shortcuts that aren't really helping you get to the finish line any faster.

Coffee. It actually just tricks your body into a false sense of sobriety. You'll be wide awake to endure the hangover though, so there's that.

Pain relievers. Your preferred over-the-counter anti-inflammatory can temporarily relieve your headache or other body aches, but it's only scratching the surface. If you're feeling really awful, stay clear of pain relievers like Tylenol. Ibuprofen (think Advil, Motrin, etc.) can cause serious damage to your body if taken in tandem with particularly large amounts of alcohol or when combined on a regular basis. Some health risks include kidney damage, gastrointestinal bleeding, lack of alertness, and less overall effectiveness of what the medication is intended for.[2] All of this is on top of the beating you just put your liver through.

Cold showers. They're good for one thing: cooling down after a day at the beach. Otherwise, you're just asking to be freezing during and shivering after. And you were trying to get rid of the shakes.

Greasy food. You may be under the impression that a bacon double cheeseburger and a side of loaded tots is going to magically soak up last night's slosh fest, but your body has already absorbed the alcohol. Satisfying our body's oddball craving for whatever's deep fried and weighed down in unhealthy fats is only going to further bury that six-pack you're working to uncover. Not that all the booze last night helped. Instead, opt for food high in nutritional value. It may not make you salivate as much as corn dogs and chili fries, but your body will appreciate the courtesy.

> **"**
> The only thing that will heal a hangover is time.

Here's the truth: The only thing that will heal a hangover is time. Your body needs that to process the alcohol it's consumed. But there's a catch. Even though time will eventually make you feel less gross, it doesn't diminish any of the work your body still has to do to get you past last night, nor will it "cure" or prevent the potential health risks that come from continued overuse and misuse.

LIFE IS TOO SHORT TO FORGET WHAT HAPPENED LAST NIGHT

MEMORIES

...and then everything went dark. "What happened last night?" Ever wake up and you can't remember how you got home? You check your phone and wish you didn't? Your heart pulses with anxiety as you scroll through a thread of texts from your friends wondering where you went or if you're okay. Your replies are all consonants, no vowels. Your timeline

> **"**
> 'What happened last night?'
> You blacked out.

shows that you checked into three bars you swear you've never been to. And, when you nervously look at your photos, you realize that you sent one of *those pics*. You blacked out.

That hazy feeling after drinking too much alcohol is actually because it's affected a part of the brain called the hippocampus, which helps us form, process, and retrieve two types of memories: declarative and spatial relationship. These memories are related to facts and events, and involve pathways or routes, respectively. It's there in our brain where short-term memories are then locked into long-term ones.[3] This is why after a night of heavy or binge drinking it's sometimes difficult to recall certain events, or the entire night. We believe in creating awesome memories from amazing experiences, and *remembering* them. Drinking too much can easily prevent that from happening. It steals experiences and time we can't ever get back.

Lost memories from heavy drinking can also have serious consequences on your ability to learn and retain information. Unfortunately, it's not as simple as just not drinking when you're studying. Memory formation is a complex process that develops over time. Much of what you're trying to commit to memory from class is solidified when you're not thinking about the material. In fact, much of memory formation occurs while you sleep, and alcohol dramatically affects your sleep cycle.

> **"**
> We believe in creating awesome memories from amazing experiences, and *remembering* them.

SLEEP

Passing out is not the same as falling asleep naturally.

And going to one more bar to have a nightcap because it sounds sexy is not helping you once your head hits the pillow. Our body's sleep/wake cycle is conditioned by a 24-hour internal clock, known as our circadian rhythm, that tick-tocks within the brain's hypothalamus. That rhythm is most in tune when we adhere to a regular sleep schedule.

Alcohol is one of the most common, yet ill-advised, sleep aids. It should not be considered an option. Yes, it brings on sleepiness and induces sleep, but it forces our body to nod off to an offbeat drummer and diminishes those high quality and peaceful Z's. Over time, alcohol used as a crutch to help you fall asleep, or consumed in place of what would be your normal bedtime, can cause insomnia by interfering with the body's built-in system for regulating sleep. "Alcohol suppresses breathing and can precipitate sleep apnea" (i.e., pauses/disruptions in breathing during sleep), says Irshaad Ebrahim, medical director at The London Sleep Centre.[4] Even drinking recreationally as far as three to six hours before you go to bed can disrupt the sequence and duration of normal sleep, reducing your brain's ability to retain any information you learned earlier that day.

> **"**
> Alcohol is one of the most common, yet ill-advised, sleep aids.

Stages of REM and deep sleep are crucial for cognition and memory, and essential for sleep to feel restorative, says Dr. Rajkumar Dasgupta, assistant professor at the University of Southern California's Keck School of Medicine.[5] You may think that because that last drink at last call made you zonk out in a flash earned you a solid night's sleep, but what you probably don't realize or remember are the times throughout the night that the alcohol in your system robbed you of sleeping soundly. Michael Breus, PhD, clinical psychologist, Diplomate of the American Board of Sleep Medicine, and Fellow of The American Academy of Sleep Medicine, warns that alcohol-influenced sleep creates a greater likelihood to sleepwalk, sleep talk, and sleep eat, among other zombie-like behaviors.[6]

> **"**
> The alcohol in your system robbed you of sleeping soundly.

PERFORMANCE

Wakey, wakey! Time for eggs and bakey! Hey, rise and shine! Oh, too loud? Too early? C'mon, outta bed! It's literally after noon. It's going to be a long one because hangovers can sometimes seem to linger for days. Being lazily idle from feeling lethargic can compound into a physical drag on your A game. Unless, of course, there's a trophy for binge-watching Netflix in your sweats.

> ACADEMIC PERFORMANCE

Balancing a full class load can be stressful enough as it is. Waking up feeling like death from a hangover isn't going to help. You'll only be able to skip class so many times before you become a "Fifth Year." The Harvard School of Public Health found that one in four college students admit academic consequences from drinking, including missing class, falling behind in class, doing poorly on papers or exams, and receiving lower grades overall.[7]

Do you know what the difference is between being book smart and street smart? It's the learning curve that connects knowledge and experience. This book hopes to shorten that distance

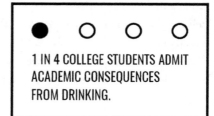

1 IN 4 COLLEGE STUDENTS ADMIT ACADEMIC CONSEQUENCES FROM DRINKING.

for anyone who lacks either, but thinks they know better. You don't have to read this book for the following truths to make sense. However, underestimating the likelihood that we could become a statistic if we don't slow our drinking may result in us learning a lesson the hard way. It's a myth that we have to personally endure failure or pain and suffering as a prerequisite to learn from experience.

> ATHLETIC PERFORMANCE

If you're an athlete or someone who values the achievement from physical activity or sports, you should be extra cautious about your alcohol intake. Curling more pitchers of beer than weights will set you back in your training, on game day, and during recovery.

Alcohol disrupts your body's ability to absorb protein, impacting protein synthesis that helps you build

ATTENDANCE

Frequency of alcohol consumption was associated positively with absenteeism from classes disliked.[8]

28%

Alcohol is a factor in 28% of college dropouts.[9]

STUDYING

There is a negative relationship between heavy episodic alcohol use and the time students spend on academics.[10]

  More than one-third of binge drinkers report falling behind in their schoolwork due to drinking.[11]

GPA

The probability of getting a high GPA significantly decreases as the frequency of heavy episodic drinking increases.[12]

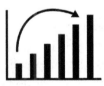

Binge drinkers are six times more likely than those who drink but don't binge to perform poorly on a test or project.[13]

The heaviest drinkers obtain the lowest grades.[14]

Alcohol consumption has a negative predictive effect on GPA under all definitions of drinking (binge, frequent binge, drunkenness, and frequent drunkenness).[15]

> **"**
> It's a myth that we have to personally endure failure or pain and suffering as a prerequisite to learn from experience.

muscle. You've already read that alcohol interrupts a good night's sleep, during which an important chemical called human growth hormone (hGH) is released. hGH is vital in the growth and repair of your muscles, but alcohol can decrease the secretion of hGH by as much as 70%.[16]

Alcohol lowers testosterone. The presence of alcohol in your body triggers a multitude of chemical processes, including the release of a toxin from your liver that attacks the amount of testosterone you have.

Alcohol is a diuretic, which increases the need to go to the bathroom, and thus contributes to dehydration. We all end up breaking the seal. In turn, dehydration leads to greater risk of sustaining musculoskeletal injuries such as cramps and muscle strains.

Oh yeah, alcohol is also pretty unforgiving in packing on the pounds, too. Did you really think putting on the "Freshman 15" was exclusive to underclassmen? Alcohol is empty calories—meaning they provide no nutritional value. An average light beer contains over 100 calories. A glass of wine? A few more than that. A Long Island Iced Tea? You don't even want to know. You could easily be drinking a very unhealthy and hefty meal during a night out without even realizing it.

> "
> Alcohol consumption increases fat storage and can adversely affect your percentage of body fat.

Alcohol reduces the amount of fat our body burns for energy. Our muscles aren't able to use these calories for fuel, so instead of being converted to glycogen (a form of stored carbohydrates), our body treats alcohol as fat. As a result, alcohol consumption increases fat storage and can adversely affect your percentage of body fat.

Conveniently enough, alcohol also stimulates appetite. So that large pizza with an extra side of ranch delivered to your apartment at 3 a.m. to cushion the last few drinks will not only show up tomorrow in the mirror and on the scale, it's going to weigh you down on the field or court, too. Heavy drinking in the midst of needing to rely on your body's physical abilities is essentially taking one step

> "
> The intellectual and physical toll that drinking can have on the body is obvious and recognizable, but the long-term effects can be severe and irreversible.

forward and two steps back, which is ironically how you'd probably walk when you've had too much to drink.

The intellectual and physical toll that drinking can have on the body is obvious and recognizable, but the long-term effects can be severe and irreversible. The party last night might've been next level, but it could keep you on the bench and stunt your chances to get (or keep) that academic or athletic scholarship.

WE ENCOURAGE CHOICES THAT REDUCE OUR RISK FOR ADDICTION

DEPENDENCY AND ADDICTION

Not becoming dependent on or addicted to alcohol can preserve our long-term relationship with it. Assuming we enter a relationship with alcohol with a clean slate (i.e., a healthy, stable, and capable mind and body), we become the masters of our own free will. Albeit, we must acknowledge that we're up against constricting pressure to look, feel, and act like one of the cool kids. Conversely, we also have to accept ownership and responsibility for our own decisions.

If you'd like to spend your life enjoying a healthy relationship with alcohol, then you should drink in a way that will lower your risk for substance use disorder or, specifically, alcohol use disorder (AUD). AUD is a chronic relapsing brain disease characterized by compulsive alcohol use—an impaired ability to stop or control alcohol use

> **"**
> Not becoming dependent on or addicted to alcohol can preserve our long-term relationship with it.

despite adverse social, occupational, or health consequences.[17] Although addiction is complicated, researchers have identified four major risk factors that contribute to a person's susceptibility to it: genetics, age, consumption behavior, and psychological and environmental circumstances.

RISK FACTORS

> GENETICS

The reality, for some of us, is that we have to consider the hand we're dealt. The *Center on Addiction* finds that 50-75% of a person's predisposition to addiction can be linked to genetic factors.[18] By no fault of our own, we might simply be more at risk of becoming addicted if we have an immediate blood relative who struggles with addiction. It's important to talk with your parents about whether anyone in your family has had a history with alcohol or substance abuse to determine if you are potentially at greater risk. Children of parents with alcohol dependence or AUD are four to 10 times more likely to become challenged with

> **"**
> 50-75% of a person's predisposition to addiction can be linked to genetic factors.

dependence themselves or develop AUD than children who do not have close relatives with problematic alcohol use.[19] Should you have that conversation with a loved one, do so with empathy and grace. There is no need to embarrass or shame them.

> AGE

There is a significant amount of research and evidence that shows the younger an individual is when he or she starts drinking, the greater the likelihood for addiction and potential damage to the brain. The reason is because our brain is still developing, which makes it much more sensitive to the effects and impact of alcohol. In the forthcoming section, *Why wait?*, we explain why patience is a virtue.

> CONSUMPTION BEHAVIOR

Addiction to alcohol can be fueled by the euphoric effects associated with over-consuming and getting drunk. Repeatedly drinking past the point of feeling buzzed can be foreshadowing that you're heading down a slippery slope. In doing so, your body is going to build up its tolerance to alcohol,

> **"**
> The younger an individual is when he or she starts drinking, the greater the likelihood for addiction and potential damage to the brain.

which raises the bar for how much you'll have to drink next time to chase the same buzz. Drinking in moderation does a body good by not subjecting it to the onslaught of risky consequences from over-intoxication.

> PSYCHOLOGICAL AND ENVIRONMENTAL CIRCUMSTANCES

Stress, anxiety, and depression as well as personality tendencies that lean toward high impulsivity or the pressing itch for sensation gratification can blur the lines between clear, rational, safe decisions. Emotional, physical, or sexual abuse or trauma may also lead to survivors attempting to cope or numb the pain by self-medicating. Ease of access to alcohol, and a bombardment from media and marketing that encourages gluttonous consumption without consequence are also contributing factors to an increased risk for addiction. If we're not careful, drinking while under duress or at the mercy of our environment can exasperate veiled problems and expedite alcohol's subtle way of sneaking up on us, and set us up for failure.

ALCOHOL SHOULD BE A CRAFT THAT'S ENJOYED— NOT A TOOL FOR DEALING WITH LIFE

The more risk factors present, the greater your chance for dependency and addiction. This does not mean that we are automatically prone to addiction should any apply; however, the presence of these factors does raise the probability.[20] Using alcohol in an attempt to defy or circumvent an underlying core issue of an already-stacked deck will almost always ensure that the house wins. It's helpful to be able to recognize these factors in advance as well as identify the warning signs as a prelude to addiction if and when problems arise.

Persistent periods of heavy drinking can lead to a physical dependence. The first sign that you may be susceptible to addiction is an increase in tolerance. Boasting about being able to crush an entire 30 rack of the cheap stuff by yourself and "still not feel it" is not the safest or most impressive party trick.

In all seriousness, if you display multiple warning signs of dependency or full-blown addiction *(see the next page)*, it could already be, or lead to, AUD.[21]

The Recovery Village, a network of personalized rehabilitation facilities, gauges the presence of AUD if someone identifies as having at least two of these symptoms. They indicate the degree of AUD as such: mild (two to three

> **"**
> The first sign that you may be susceptible to addiction is an increase in tolerance.

symptoms), moderate (four to five), and severe (six or more).[22] Included in these are common signs of withdrawal: shaky hands, headache, nausea, sweating, vomiting, and insomnia. One in five college students meet the criteria for having AUD.[23]

Once you develop an addiction, the only form of wellness or recovery may be complete abstinence and sobriety. Even worse are some of the more severe associated dangers *(see page 50)*.

WARNING SIGNS

- Needing to drink in order to relax
- Making excuses for your drinking
- Experiencing withdrawal symptoms
- Worrying about running out of alcohol
- Lying to others about your alcohol use
- Having relationship problems due to alcohol
- Inability to concentrate due to alcohol cravings
- Having legal problems as a result of your drinking
- Drinking more as a result of a tolerance to alcohol
- Losing time from work or school due to your drinking
- Showing a lack of interest in things you once enjoyed
- Drinking more or for a longer period of time than intended
- Decreased participation in activities which were once important
- Inability to care for a family, hold down a job, or perform in school
- Feeling incapable of cutting back on the amount of alcohol consumed
- Becoming sick for an extended period of time due to drinking too much
- Finding oneself in dangerous or harmful situations as a result of drinking
- Continuing to drink despite problems with friends, family, school, or work
- Engaging in risky behaviors like unprotected sex or driving while intoxicated
- Continuing to drink despite blacking out or complicating other health problems

→ Risk of death from drunk driving (Do we even have to say this?)
→ Unintentional injuries (Dang. Where'd that bruise come from?)
→ Birth defects (Being a parent is a privilege, don't abuse it.)
→ Permanent damage to the liver, brain, and other internal organs (Thank you, but we'll go with another donor.)
→ Increased risk of certain types of cancers (Don't give the Big C a head start.)
→ Increased risk of homicide and suicide (You matter. The world needs you.)

WHY WAIT?

Waiting until you turn 21 before you consider to start drinking is one of the easiest ways to reduce your risk for AUD, addiction, and compromised biological development. Based on research from *Center on Addiction*, 96.5% of addiction cases involved people who abused substances (including alcohol) before the age of 21.[24] Further, 90% of people with an addiction to alcohol started drinking before the age of 18.[25]

Science tells us that the brain is in a high-development growth phase through our early to mid-20s. Exposing the brain to addictive substances before or during these ages leaves it much more vulnerable to coerced rewiring and the development of addiction. "Youth who start drinking before age 15 are six times

> **"**
> 96.5% of addiction cases involved people who abused substances (including alcohol) before the age of 21.

more likely to develop alcohol dependence or abuse later in life than those who begin drinking at or after age

21."[26] Expediting this forecast is that young people ages 12-20 who do drink consume more than 90% of their alcohol by binge drinking.[27]

Introducing alcohol to our bodies during this critical stage of development, especially when drinking heavily, not only affects both the brain's structure and function, but may also cause cognitive or learning problems.[28] So, if any minors in your friend network ask why they should wait until 21, your answer should be: "Drinking before you turn 21 is not healthy. It can result in impaired brain development, and it increases your risk for addiction." No, it doesn't sound appealing for a reason, but those consequences will impact your life a lot more than paying a modest fine for a misdemeanor MIP.

> "
> Drinking before you turn 21 is not healthy. It can result in impaired brain development, and it increases your risk for addiction.

2 BETTER RELATIONSHIPS

Drunk you is not the real you. It's not a better version of you, either. Some people rely on using alcohol, or worse—become dependent on it, for confidence to socialize because they haven't learned how to be comfortable without it. It's okay to be uncomfortable in navigating our journey through adolescence into adulthood. Being vulnerable means being human. Reaching for the bottle as an automatic detour around discovering who you're meant to be will undoubtedly turn you into someone you're really not. It's the unpredictable Mr. Hyde to our inherently good Dr. Jekyll. The obnoxiously intoxicated you is a false identity of who you are. It's a mask we're pressured to slip on and

> **"**
> Drunk you is
> not the real you.

hide behind to protect our insecurities, and it always makes us look less attractive than we truly are.

ALCOHOL SHOULD NEVER TURN US INTO SOMEONE WE'RE NOT

You know that one shirt you wear when you want everyone to know how much you love drinking—with the played-out, cliché boozy pun? Yeah, we see you. From a mile away. You're the life of the party—when you're drunk. You think everyone is your biggest fan. In reality, they just know to always have their thumb ready to hit *record* every time you yell, "Full send!" because you can do that thing where you smash a can of beer against your forehead repeatedly until it bursts. Hilarious. About that concussion though. At tailgating, you show off your latest wrestling moves by jumping off your truck onto a flimsy folding table, catapulting red Solo Cups everywhere. Hope you brought extra because you just spilled my drink. And you immediately want to start swingin' fists in the club because you think somebody just touched your girl. Do you *really* want to become a meme that exploits you at a low, embarrassing, regrettable moment?

Friends, we know that's not you.

Alcohol creates a distorted view of a sober reality. Don't let the initial fun buzz of your first or second drink throw you. Being impaired overrides clarity, and replaces it with shortsightedness. It alters our ability to express our feelings calmly. It also complicates social cues registering as inappropriate, which can swing our internal pendulum in opposing extremes. It causes us to act out of character and react with irrational responses. It burns bridges—some of which can never be rebuilt.

ALCOHOL SHOULD NEVER HURT RELATIONSHIPS

Going overboard with booze, even just once, can destroy relationships and cause us to drown in emotional harm. A misuse or abuse of alcohol will leave a path of indiscriminate destruction with no regard for who or what it takes out in the process. Enemy #1: ourselves. Enemy #2: everyone else.

When we dive into the behavioral effects of alcohol in *Chapter 5*, you probably won't be surprised that alcohol lowers your inhibitions. The result is a finely sharpened, double-edged sword. Quite common is how dramatically it can turn the honeymoon phase of a relationship into a fight about who gets to keep the dog and flatscreen TV. While a drink or two may initially make us relaxed and nudge us to untuck our shirt, loosen our tie, or let our hair down, a couple more can just as easily make us regret what we just said. Plainly, "Alcohol reduces our ability to think straight," says Professor McMurran, a psychologist at the University of Nottingham in the United Kingdom.[29]

Alcohol has this tricky way of fooling our brain into making us more assertive and unapologetic. You might've heard some variation of, "If you say it drunk, you mean it sober." It's because alcohol has an ill-applied reputation for being a truth serum of sorts. For relationships, especially those already on shaky ground, too much alcohol can make us vomit insensitive and spiteful words to those whom we claim to love

> **"**
> Alcohol creates a distorted view of a sober reality.

the most. Worryingly, verbal aggressiveness instigated by alcohol can amplify into domestic violence, rape, or assault. No better is the weak excuse, "But I was drunk." That's not a defense. If we do it drunk, we'll pay for it sober.

As human beings, we are equal parts strong and fragile. We have the natural born ability to tap into seemingly unnatural strength to withstand monumental challenges thrown at us. However, our emotional state is the core foundation on which our resilience is built. Depression

> **"**
> Depression and
> anxiety can be
> intensified by alcohol.

and anxiety can be intensified by alcohol. It's critical that we get our mind right before cloudy judgment deceives us into thinking that we can play with fire and not get burned. We jeopardize the health and safety of ourselves and those around us when we allow alcohol to make decisions we otherwise wouldn't when we're sober.

The emotional and physical scars left are nearly beyond comprehension. These realities can all be avoided if we put into check one common denominator: drinking *too much*. Even the most compassionate extensions of forgiveness cannot undo the gut-wrenching regret we'd feel if any of the above happened to us.

Ladies and gentlemen, we have to hold ourselves to a better standard than this, and treat each other with more decency and respect. We are worth more than the bizarro version of ourselves that an overconsumption of alcohol turns us into. When alcohol influences us to do things we wouldn't normally do, we are almost guaranteed to look in the mirror only to see someone we don't recognize staring back.

"I'm *SO* sorry." Whether you've whispered this to yourself with your head buried in your hands or swore it with the utmost sincerity between tears and sobs to your mom, best friend, or soon-to-be ex, apologizing for what you did

FOR COLLEGE STUDENTS IN PARTICULAR, THE STATISTICS ARE STAGGERING, SADDENING, AND REPREHENSIBLE.

90% of of all reported sexual assault and rape on college campuses involved the use of alcohol by the assailant, victim, or both.[30]

95% of all violent crimes on college campuses involved the use alcohol.[31]

APPROXIMATELY 696,000 STUDENT ASSAULTS PER YEAR INVOLVE ALCOHOL.[32]

Over 60% of all injuries, vandalism, and problems with the police reported on college campuses involve frequent (weekly) binge drinkers.[33]

60% of college women who have acquired sexually transmitted diseases, including HIV, were under the influence of alcohol at the time they had intercourse.[34]

when you were drunk is one of the most painful truths you'll ever confront. Okay, deep breath...

LIFE IS BETTER WITHOUT REGRETS

Did you do a tequila body shot then flash your chest for beads on spring break? Yeah, that's embarrassing. Did you ruin your buddy's wedding because you gave a drunk toast and then got asked to leave because you threw up in the country club's urinal? Been there. Did you fail out of college or get fired from your dream job because extracurricular drinking is frowned upon as professional development? Time to revise the résumé. Or botch the relationship with the one you've loved since high school because you slept with their best friend? Been there, too. We're not gonna sugarcoat it—repairing this level of damage is going to take some work. Welcome, shame. It's a notorious walk which no one should have to take.

There's a difference between crazy and stupid. University of Missouri researchers found that alcohol dulls the brain signal that warns us when we're making a mistake, ultimately reducing self-control.[35] We know this as "liquid

> Alcohol dulls the brain signal that warns us when we're making a mistake, ultimately reducing self-control.

courage"—that alcohol-induced fearlessness that can tempt us to do things that are noticeably out of character. Do not mistake your intoxicated boldness or senselessness with authentic, sober bravery. We are not heroes because others applaud our inebriated absurdity.

The embarrassment from throwing up on your roommate's cat then passing out with your shoes on to wake up as the newest member of the Pen15 club will wear—we mean wash off. The regret from missing the deadline to apply for that clutch internship won't kill you. But, when those little self-inflicted social faux pas happen over and over ... and over,

> Fair warning: there will be collateral damage.

they'll subtly start to surpass regret, harden, and solidify into shame. And, before you know it—alcohol use disorder.

Fair warning: there will be collateral damage. Shame is worse than embarrassment or regret. It's a sense of isolation from the irreversibility in knowing that an apology can't take it away. That internal, deep-to-your-core painful feeling of humiliation or distress is the consciousness of realizing that you're not in a good place. Shame is you vs. you. And both of you lose. Being humble and aware that your behavior can have dire consequences can save you from having to do emergency damage control.

3 BETTER COMMUNITIES

Contrary to what "bro-culture" party school profiles on social media try to convince you, becoming an "alcoholic" before you graduate *is* possible. You're smarter than that. Why waste those precious years getting wasted? The habits you develop while paying tens or hundreds of thousands of dollars in tuition to get an education will either follow or haunt you into adulthood.

The day after you do a cartwheel across the stage to accept your diploma, the "real world" will not wait for you to put your big boy pants on. Nor does it have the patience to tolerate your keg party antics.

You are now a fully functioning member of our free society. And we need you. Perhaps it's easy to blame our parents' or their parents' generation for the economy, environment, or lack of equality, but that doesn't mean we get to squander *our* lead. The economic burden associated with the loss of human productivity due to alcohol costs the United States approximately $250 billion a year. Yeah, with a *B*. Over three-quarters of that is related to binge drinking.[36] We don't get to say it hurts our feelings if we're contributing to that debt because quenching at Thirsty Thursdays made us call into work "sick" on Friday.

We are better served being a powerful, positive force than a threat to society. Instances of death, crime, and violence show a closely acquainted relationship with alcohol. Let's work together to advocate for better drinking which will foster healthier communities so that we can reclaim what the misuse and abuse of alcohol is expected to steal from us annually.

Alcohol is the third largest *preventable* cause of death in the United States.[37] The self-awareness that you're not producing at the level you know you're capable of due to alcohol is a powerful invitation to drink better not only for yourself, but for those around you and potentially the future branches on your family tree.

> "
> Instances of death, crime, and violence show a closely acquainted relationship with alcohol.

OVER 1,800 COLLEGE STUDENTS BETWEEN THE AGES OF 18 AND 24 DIE EVERY YEAR FROM DRINKING-RELATED CAUSES. [38]

 50%
Approximately 50% of sexual assaults involve alcohol consumption by the perpetrator, victim, or both. [39]

 40%
Alcohol is a factor in 40% of all violent crimes. [40]

 65%
65% of intimate partner violence incidents are carried out by perpetrators who've been drinking. [41]

 28%
In 2016, 28% of all traffic-related deaths in the United States involved alcohol. [42]

88,000 **PEOPLE DIE EVERY YEAR IN THE U.S. FROM ALCOHOL-RELATED CAUSES.** [43]

We want the best for you. But, living above these statistics is going to require more from us, collectively. Drinking better will have a positive domino effect where we live, play, and raise our families. You should have a fair opportunity to pursue your dreams, develop the next social network, cure cancer, or simply take an innocent walk outside without the threat of becoming a victim because you or someone else didn't know when to say, "When."

> **"**
> Drinking better
> will have a
> positive domino
> effect where we
> live, play, and
> raise our families.

Regardless of what legacy you want to leave behind, in the meantime you'll be living next to someone else and paying taxes somewhere. It's up to you whether your neighbors invite you over for a BBQ or put up a fence.

PART 2

BETTER
DRINKING
CULTURE

We believe in better drinking. If you glossed over the *Introduction* and missed where we defined what that means to us, allow us to reiterate. It's the nuts and bolts of what we're all about. Like with anything we do or care about, drinking deserves our attention and respect. To drink better is to consciously approach alcohol with mindfulness—considerate forethought and deliberate intentionality. Drinking mindfully allows us to become more aware of how our body and mind are affected by alcohol.

If you choose to have a relationship with alcohol, you should be the one who gets to call the shots. Not the guy who's already had one too many. When we lose control of ourselves because we've allowed the alcohol to order another round, the wheels fall off the bus, we start sliding, and the bus eventually slams into the guardrail. What, when, why, and how much you choose to drink is on you. If you keep those factors in check and within your own personal limits, the wheels stay on the bus.

THE R WORD

Responsibly. This might be one of the only times you ever catch us using the *R* word. In fact, you'll never hear us tell you to, "Please drink *responsibly.*" It's like a four-letter word at BDC. We cringe every time we hear it.

Dear parents, Mr. University, and the alcohol industry—if you're reading this, stay with us.

We do believe that the *R* word, particularly when attached to that seemingly sincere request, originated with good intentions. It started to appear in advertising campaigns in the 1970s; however, a *lot* has changed since then. Yet, and perhaps unknowingly, this petition in fine print now comes off as a hollow obligation. Perceptive consumers recognize that it's rather vague, leaving it up to interpretation. And, the really clever ones already have or will continue to figure out a way to drink "responsibly" around their school, work, or social responsibilities.

In fact, it can also be construed as though all problems arising from *not* drinking "responsibly" are the consumers' fault. Lawyers can sleep well at night because there's a tiny warning on a bottle or at the end of a commercial aimed at the public that told them so. This, friends, is a sliver of what's referred to as "corporate social responsibility." This worldwide initiative, which always comes *after* the alcohol is promoted, is easier and cheaper to keep rehashing than applying those efforts to educate toward a higher standard of cultural behaviors and expectations. Frankly, the R word is outdated, overused, and the impact of its original intent has been diluted to the point of misinterpretation and mockery.

New school drinkers seem to be unfazed by its presence. We know you're savvy and won't buy something just because it's being sold to you, even if it's endorsed by the pop culture influencer of the month. We've been told by countless college-age consumers that when they're exposed to the R word they either completely ignore it or consider it a green light to drink as much as they want as long as they get a "safe" ride home.

While we strongly oppose driving under the influence, the implied license to go as hard as you want when you're out drinking because you're just a couple app clicks away from a "safe" ride doesn't address the core problem. We believe the promotion of "safe rides," which is often the emphasis of "drink responsibly," might be unintentionally promoting excessive consumption. Spilling out of your preferred rideshare service or chauffeured party bus onto your doorstep only gets you home. But, you're the one who has to deal with everything that happened before you clicked *Request Ride* as well as whatever messy aftermath you might wake up to tomorrow, including being hit with that $100 fine because someone had to clean up your puke. A sober driver doesn't excuse a wasted passenger.

ALCOHOL SHOULD BE A CHOICE—NOT AN EXPECTATION

Do you think it's effective? That's not rhetorical. It's time we demand more. It's time to drink *better* because we know what *that* means.

Repeat after me: *Alcohol should be a choice—not an expectation.* If your friends jumped off of a bridge, would you do it, too? Yeah, we just went there so you don't have to. Not conforming is an option, a commendable decision when made. We sacrifice a piece of our own identity every time we yield to social pressure to fit in because it's what the in-crowd deems as popular. Instead, click *Unfollow*.

BDC's co-founder has never tasted a drop of alcohol in his life, and he's comfortable in his own sober skin. On the other hand, BDC's CEO favors double IPAs, two fingers of bourbon, and Brunello di Montalcino. And, you know what? They're still able to hang out together, eat together, and drink (whatever they choose) together because they respect each other's decision.

There's more to friendship and camaraderie than feeling obligated to be intoxicated in someone else's presence. There's nothing wrong with meeting your friends for a drink or hanging out over a couple after work. There's also nothing wrong with having an honest, deep conversation with another human without being under the influence. And while these two examples are not mutually exclusive, getting to a level with your friends that allows you the safe space to share meaningful, real experiences and be vulnerable without the presence of alcohol is truly beautiful, and will make your relationships that much more valuable. Be yourself and you will find your people.

Mindful drinking is all about deciding what's right for *you*. No one else. No matter what. We have to abandon the social norm that says drinking is just what you do—that you have to get drunk to party or have a good time. Saying, "Thanks, but I'm not drinking tonight" should not make the DJ's needle scratch. Nor should we shine an interrogation lamp at the non-drinker and make them explain themselves as if they've been accused of a crime. Unless they volunteer why, it's none of our business, so please don't ask.

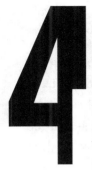

KNOW YOURSELF

Hey, what's your number? No, we're not hitting on you, but you do seem like a catch. We're asking, "Do you know what your drink limit is?" We'll get more into this in the next chapter, but, for general intents and purposes, knowing what your tolerance is up front can save you the headache of dealing with a hangover on the back end.

We understand, however, that this could be a catch-22 for anyone who has yet to drink or develop a trusted relationship with alcohol. Our journey with it starts with our first drink, and continues to adjust based on our decisions with each subsequent choice. Still, ascending from novice to expert does not imply that you have to learn by mistake or realize that you've climbed too high too fast. Know your number, and stick to it—even if your number is 0. For some it is or may need to be, and that's okay.

Self-awareness is an underutilized, powerful characteristic. However, we're bombarded from every direction by a culture that thrives on gluttonous consumption.

> **"**
> Do you know what your drink limit is?

That, unfortunately, leaves little room in our bellies to slow down long enough to think about who we are in the moment, appreciate what we're drinking, and assess why we do it to the point of needing to purge.

Being mindful means being intentional. Before you pour your first drink, set some rules for yourself, and make a plan. Note to self: The ability to strategize deteriorates *after* you're tipsy. So, consider the following in advance:

Are you going to drink? If you're making the decision based on *anyone* else, you're relinquishing control that you should be in charge of.

What is your motivation for drinking? Getting back at your ex is not a good answer.

Will drinking right now interrupt your rhythm? Are you trying to achieve a fitness goal? Do you need to make rent? How 'bout that term paper due on Monday?

Can you enjoy the occasion without a drink in your hand? You have the strength to overcome any anxiety you think will be a result of not being inebriated. Embrace the awkwardness, then you do you. Own the dance floor.

Eat. Having food in your stomach, particularly proteins, fats, and carbs, slows the absorption of alcohol into the bloodstream. Order that Buddha bowl. Intentionally avoiding eating for the conservation of calories, known as drunkorexia, is unhealthy and dangerous. It can also lead to overeating later (in the night). You're beautiful just the way you are.

How much *should* you consume? Think carefully about what your personal limit is. If you don't know, it's smart to start in first gear. Going from zero to sixty in less than three seconds is going to result in an expensive accident.

Where will you be going? *(See Chapter 6.)* If your friends ask if you want to hang out, your answer should not depend on whether there's an open bar or if you can sneak in a flask.

Will you be behind the wheel? Golf carts and riding lawn mowers included. Bicycles doubly so.

Are you pregnant, on any meds, struggling with depression or anxiety, or taking recreational drugs? We're not doctors, but if your answer to any of them is, "Yes," understand that it is not safe or recommended to mix them. Seriously.

#mood. What kind are you in? What kind do you want to avoid? How much you drink (sometimes even if it's "just one") can either maintain it or cause it to spin out of control. Even the "fun drunk" can unintentionally turn into the sad clown.

When will you stop drinking (today/tonight)? Have an exit strategy.

What obligations or commitments do you have later tonight or tomorrow morning? Even if you think your answer is, "Nada," your default answer should always be, "Myself."

In the whole grand scheme of things, your well-being is invariably important. The health of your mental and emotional state may, in fact, be the single most significant consideration in how (or whether) you should approach a relationship with alcohol, if at all, or continue that relationship. While alcohol may be used to "take the edge off," the relief is temporary. The first few sips can do that, but those edges will continue to become more jagged over time. Alcohol can just as much elevate our mood in a positive direction as it can stop on a dime without notice, and drag us 180° in the opposite direction toward a really bad one. Drinking as a coping mechanism to escape—to express, mask, or avoid feelings—is not healthy, but all too common.

This certainly comes with a perplexing challenge. In particular, depression and AUD have a causal relationship. Although a study in *Addiction* found that alcohol abuse is more likely to cause major depression than the other way around, it also points out that the causality could go in either direction.[44] In essence, alcohol abuse can result in depression just as depression can result in alcohol abuse. Nearly one-third of people with clinical depression experience problems associated with

> **"**
> Alcohol abuse is more likely to *cause* major depression than the other way around.

their drinking.[45] Those struggling with either affliction often find themselves caught in a vicious cycle that may appear to have no end because its starting point may have been a blurry, moving target in the first place. Breaking that cycle may seem impossible for those who are stuck spinning within it. Although this is a battle many people often (think they have to) fight alone, help and treatment are available. Overcoming these challenges is aided by healthy support from friends, family, professionals, and those who care. Let the right people in who can help shine light on the darkness.

5 KNOW YOUR DRINK

Alcohol is obviously an intoxicant, yet dually a depressant. This complicates things before we even begin. While we often thrive on chasing its socially euphoric effects, over-consumption of alcohol can tip the scales and drag us to a dark place. By nature, the characteristic dichotomy of alcohol's makeup can be a recipe for disaster so we need to know the ingredients we're working with.

In its simplest terms, the alcohol we drink is the result of fermentation—a biological process induced by yeast that converts sugars into energy, producing ethanol (i.e., ethyl alcohol or pure alcohol) and carbon dioxide as by-products. Pure alcohol is what causes intoxication.

As a snapshot of most of the types of alcohol commonly consumed, beer is produced by fermentation of grain starches. Spirits (i.e., liquor) pick up where beer leaves off with the additional process of distillation. Wine, cider, and perry are produced by the fermentation of natural sugars found in grapes, apples, and pears. And mead is produced by fermentation of the natural sugars

> **"**
> Not all alcoholic beverages are created equal, but they all contain pure alcohol.

present in honey. Not all alcoholic beverages are created equal, but they all contain pure alcohol.

ABV

Alcohol by volume (ABV) is the universally recognized standard measure of how much alcohol (ethanol) is contained in a given volume of an alcoholic beverage (expressed as a volume percent). In the U.S., it's common for the alcohol strength of spirits to be listed as "proof" rather than ABV, which is essentially twice the alcohol by volume. For example, typical vodka that's 40% ABV will likely read as 80 proof on its label.

STANDARD DRINK EQUIVALENTS

The U.S. Department of Health and Human Services' Dietary Guidelines for Americans (DGA) defines one "standard drink" by the following equivalents, each of which contains about a ½ oz (15 ml) of pure alcohol.[46]

BEER
12 oz (355 ml)
5% ABV

WINE
5 oz (128 ml)
12% ABV

SPIRITS
1.5 oz (44 ml)
80 proof

Keep in mind, these standards get thrown out the window as soon as variables are introduced. Depending on what your drink of choice is, its strength, the volume you consume, and the rate at which you do all play a key role in how your night will play out. The DGA calculates drink equivalents of selected beverages as such:

DRINK EQUIVALENTS

BEER

12 fl oz at 4.2% (a typical, popular "light" beer)	0.8
12 fl oz at 5% (reference beverage)	1
16 fl oz at 5%	1.3
12 fl oz at 7%	1.4
12 fl oz at 9%	1.8

WINE

5 fl oz at 12% (reference beverage)	1
9 fl oz at 12%	1.8
5 fl oz at 15%	1.3
5 fl oz at 17%	1.4

SPIRITS

1.5 fl oz 80 proof spirits (40%) (reference beverage)	1
Mixed drinks with more than 1.5 fl oz 80 proof spirits (40%)	>1

To calculate drink equivalents, multiply the volume in ounces by the alcohol content in percent and divide by 0.6 ounces of alcohol per drink equivalent. For example, 16 oz of beer at 5% is calculated as (16 oz)(0.05)/0.6 oz = 1.3 drink equivalents.

Depending on the type of spirits and a cocktail's other ingredients, one mixed drink can contain a variable number of drink equivalents. Carbonated mixers like tonic water, soda/pop, etc. speed up alcohol absorption. When it comes to sophisticated mixed cocktails or anything that's served in a fishbowl, there's no hard and fast rule to determine how much pure alcohol you're getting. Don't be afraid to ask your server or bartender about what you're ordering. A professional mixologist should be able to tell you at least what liquor is in the recipe as well as strength and volume of each, but then you might have to do the math on your own. If your "drink" requires a minimum number of people to order it, two hands to hold, shows up with a handful of straws, a pound of gummi bears as its garnish, and is then set on fire, all bets are off.

BAC

The amount of ethanol in the body is quantified by blood alcohol content (BAC), which is weight of ethanol per unit volume of blood. Ingesting alcohol in small, manageable amounts gives us the stimulant-like warm fuzzies we enjoy from drinking. However, those feelings can go south quickly when we consume more alcohol than our bodies can handle.

APPROXIMATE BAC CALCULATOR

The chart on the next page is based on a person's sex, body weight, and the number of "standard" drinks consumed. It does not take into account variable intoxication rate factors that affect alcohol absorption (e.g., rate of consumption, food intake, drug use, body size, body fat, etc.), all of which can affect BAC. For example, women tend to become intoxicated faster than men, even if they're of similar body weight and drinking equivalent amounts at the same pace. Because women absorb and metabolize alcohol differently due to having less body water and more body fat than men, they achieve higher concentrations of alcohol in the blood and thus reach a higher BAC quicker.[47]

Typically, our bodies require approximately one hour to process one standard drink from our system. Nothing can speed up this process. It's also to be noted that just because you stop drinking

> **"**
> Typically, our bodies require approximately one hour to process one standard drink from our system. Nothing can speed up this process.

doesn't mean your BAC has stopped rising. Absorption continues from 30 to 90 minutes after you've actually stopped drinking, depending on how much food has been consumed as well as other intoxication rate factors that may contribute to this equation.

DRINKS	SEX	BODY WEIGHT (lb)								
		90	100	120	140	160	180	200	220	240
1	Male	—	.04	.03	.03	.02	.02	.02	.02	.02
	Female	.05	.05	.04	.03	.03	.03	.02	.02	.02
2	Male	—	.08	.06	.05	.05	.04	.04	.03	.03
	Female	.10	.09	.08	.07	.06	.05	.05	.04	.04
3	Male	—	.11	.09	.08	.07	.06	.06	.05	.05
	Female	.15	.14	.11	.10	.09	.08	.07	.06	.06
4	Male	—	.15	.12	.11	.09	.08	.08	.07	.06
	Female	.20	.18	.15	.13	.11	.10	.09	.08	.08
5	Male	—	.19	.16	.13	.12	.11	.09	.09	.08
	Female	.25	.23	.19	.16	.14	.13	.11	.10	.09
6	Male	—	.23	.19	.16	.14	.13	.11	.10	.09
	Female	.30	.27	.23	.19	.17	.15	.14	.12	.11
7	Male	—	.26	.22	.19	.16	.15	.13	.12	.11
	Female	.35	.32	.27	.23	.20	.18	.16	.14	.13
8	Male	—	.30	.25	.21	.19	.17	.15	.14	.13
	Female	.40	.36	.30	.26	.23	.20	.18	.17	.15
9	Male	—	.34	.28	.24	.21	.19	.17	.15	.14
	Female	.45	.41	.34	.29	.26	.23	.20	.19	.17
10	Male	—	.38	.31	.27	.23	.21	.19	.17	.16
	Female	.51	.45	.38	.32	.28	.25	.23	.21	.19

This chart should not be used as a scientific tool or an exact system of measurememt.

When a person's BAC escalates into extremely dangerous ranges, life threatening consequences from severe intoxication become imminent.

BAC up to 0.3% can result in confusion, aggression, and a diminished ability to feel pain. Even higher BAC up to 0.4% can result in lapses in and out of consciousness, becoming incapacitated, and the inability to become aroused. Finally, as BAC level approaches 0.5%, a person can die from a variety of physiological complications including slowing heart rate, lower respiration, diminished reflexes, and decreased body temperature. It's to be noted that death may occur at 0.37% or higher, and BAC levels of 0.45% and higher are fatal to almost everyone.[48]

BINGE DRINKING DEFINED

The definition of binge drinking is defined differently, however similarly, by various institutions. Two often-referenced measures include:

"A pattern of drinking that brings blood alcohol content (BAC) levels to 0.08. Typically, this occurs after four drinks for women and five drinks for men—in two hours." National Institute on Alcohol Abuse and Alcoholism (NIAAA)

"When men consume five or more [standard] drinks, and women consume four or more [standard] drinks, within a two-hour period." Substance Abuse and Mental Health

Services Administration (SAMHSA)

Now that we understand how a standard drink is defined, it helps put the formal definition of binge drinking into context. These parameters are justified in establishing a baseline, but its significance can't be measured in absolutes. Binge drinking should be recognized through a wider lens, particularly when drinking heavily socially.

It's probably safe to assume that when most people hear the term "binge drinking" they don't automatically calculate their consumption in terms of number of drinks by timeframe. Rather, we tend to think of it in its simplest identifiable characteristics: deliberately drinking more than what would otherwise be considered safe, resulting in over-intoxication and potentially dangerous consequences.

Regardless of how *you* define it, you're smart enough to know that binge drinking has an overwhelmingly negative connotation for good reason. Yet, we call it "partying" because it sounds cooler and less self-inflicting, and we keep on chuggin' along like it can't touch us. But it does. Sooner or later, in some form, it will catch up to us. Embracing a lifestyle of drinking better can undoubtedly save you from carrying the heavy weight of shame and regret that typically goes hand in hand with drinking just to get hammered-drunk.

> **"**
> Embracing a lifestyle of drinking better can undoubtedly save you from carrying the heavy weight of shame and regret that typically goes hand in hand with drinking just to get hammered-drunk.

ALCOHOL POISONING

Alcohol poisoning is an understood threat of binge drinking. On average, six people die every day in the U.S. from it.[49] It occurs when alcohol is consumed faster than the body can absorb and process it. Alcohol poisoning commonly happens in conjunction with being challenged to drink on a bet or dare. What's particularly dangerous about rapid binge drinking is that you're physically able to consume a fatal dose of alcohol before your body loses consciousness. Alcohol impairs our central nervous system.

LIFE-THREATENING SIGNS OF ALCOHOL POISONING[50]

- Inability to wake up
- Vomiting
- Slow breathing (fewer than eight breaths per minute)
- Irregular breathing (10 seconds or more between breaths)
- Seizures
- Hypothermia (low body temperature), bluish skin color, paleness

Dear friends,

When someone tries to intervene to help that wobbly person who's clearly had too much to drink, please don't tell everyone, "No, it's cool. He's not driving." That's not an acceptable answer. Just because they're not behind the wheel does not mean they're in the clear from how much they've consumed. Because our BAC can continue to rise even while unconscious, "taking care of" our friends by putting them to bed or letting them pass out on the couch so they can "sleep it off" may actually be putting them in serious danger. If you ever suspect someone is at risk of alcohol poisoning, call 911 immediately. Pride and ego are <u>not</u> more valuable than someone's life.

WE EMBRACE QUALITY OVER QUANTITY

Raise your hand if you've ever started pre-partying with your buddies and declared, "LET'S GET F-ING WASTED TONIGHT!" Keep your hand up if on Sunday morning you've jumped out of bed before noon screaming, "Hangovers are my favorite! I'm going to be able to accomplish so much today!" Nah, we didn't think so. You don't get to have both. Interestingly enough, we've never heard, "I'm SO stoked to go out binge drinking this weekend!" It just doesn't have quite the same ring to it, does it? But, if we had a dime for every time we've heard, "Ugh... I am N E V E R drinking again," we'd own Amazon, or Apple, or both. It takes less energy, time, and money to remember last night than it does to forget it.

It's not about drinking just for the sake of drinking, but more about how you *experience* it. Respecting the craft (and the substance as a chemical) means appreciating everything about the lifecycle that went into what you're consuming: from how it's made to how it ended up in the glass in front of you. It also includes all of the talented people who had a hand in making it happen.

In this context, *craft* is not meant to be synonymous with *local* or *independent*, but the artform. It reflects the skill of what it took to bring that beverage to life in order for you to enjoy it. Regardless of what your drink of choice is, own it. What you're drinking is backed by sweat equity. It's a work of art and should be treated as such. Your parents don't spend all day preparing Thanksgiving dinner for the entire family only to watch you scarf it down without coming up for air. Slow down, take a breath, pace yourself, and savor what's in front of you. The drinking experience can and should be about more than the sheer volume of what you can put down.

BEHAVIORAL EFFECTS

It's important to understand that a person's tolerance does not affect their BAC, nor is it always a reliable indicator of how intoxicated they are or seem. Tolerance only masks how drunk you *appear*. It does not mean you'll pass that breathalyzer when the blues and reds are in your rearview mirror—even if you think you're "fine." And just because you can "hold" your booze better than others doesn't mean you'll be immune to its negative side effects.

ALCOHOL SHOULD NEVER PUT OURSELVES OR OTHERS IN HARM'S WAY

For some, even a single drink will alter a person's behavior. The time it takes for a person to "feel" the effects of alcohol can vary. Considering intoxication rate factors can help you assess how quickly you might feel alcohol "kick in." Depending on what factors are applicable, it could be as soon as 10 minutes or as long as 90. The keyword here is *patience*. Allow time for

> "
> A person's tolerance does not affect their BAC. Tolerance only masks how drunk you *appear*.

what you've just consumed to metabolize through your body. If you wait long enough between drinks (have a water while you're at it) you'll be better able to gauge how it affects your body. Generally speaking, the more alcohol there is in your bloodstream, the more obvious the following cues will be *(see the next page)*.

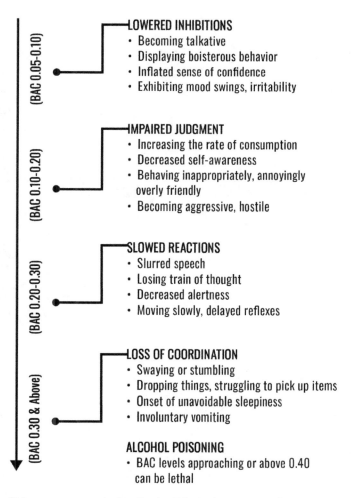

(BAC 0.05-0.10)

LOWERED INHIBITIONS
- Becoming talkative
- Displaying boisterous behavior
- Inflated sense of confidence
- Exhibiting mood swings, irritability

(BAC 0.10-0.20)

IMPAIRED JUDGMENT
- Increasing the rate of consumption
- Decreased self-awareness
- Behaving inappropriately, annoyingly overly friendly
- Becoming aggressive, hostile

(BAC 0.20-0.30)

SLOWED REACTIONS
- Slurred speech
- Losing train of thought
- Decreased alertness
- Moving slowly, delayed reflexes

(BAC 0.30 & Above)

LOSS OF COORDINATION
- Swaying or stumbling
- Dropping things, struggling to pick up items
- Onset of unavoidable sleepiness
- Involuntary vomiting

ALCOHOL POISONING
- BAC levels approaching or above 0.40 can be lethal

BAC ranges are approximate estimates. Behavioral cues can vary from person to person. Any speculation of one's BAC or speculated correlation between these behavioral cues and one's BAC should not be assumed.

6 KNOW YOUR ENVIRONMENT

Lock it up. Getting plastered should not be a requirement in order to have fun. We're not so naive as to ignore the undeniable role that alcohol does play in enhancing an already enjoyable experience. For some, perhaps, it creates an *illusion* of enhancement. Nonetheless, we're certainly not going to be hypocrites who say we've never drank and had a good time at the same time. Again, the two are not mutually exclusive. Moreso, don't let your brain's buzz fool you into believing that the potential for the amount of fun you can have must correlate to an increased alcohol intake.

> **"**
> Getting plastered
> should not be a
> requirement in order
> to have fun.

Remember what it was like being a kid? We could have all the fun in the world. Sober. But, as adults, we tend to forget what that childlike innocence felt like, and we get trapped into the habit of using alcohol to unlock a bonus level of fun that we discredit as being unattainable without being cocktailed up. We have to refuse to accept the idea that being sober is boring. It's tough, because alcohol is so ingrained in our culture's very spirited history. Establishing a few common and low-maintenance practices can help us ride the wave of a perfect buzz without crashing into the shore headfirst.

Identifying that sweet spot can be like finding a needle in a haystack. We're all looking for our own—that relatively narrow window where we feel connected and relaxed, yet still in control of our thoughts and behavior. One sip too

> **"**
> We have to refuse to
> accept the idea that
> being sober is boring.

many, and we lose our balance and wipe out. Honing in on the right amount to drink—for you, on your terms—does not have to be an elusive mirage.

Reference *Chapter 4* for making a plan before your drinking session commences. Once it's started, add these skills to your repertoire to stay in control. *No one* likes a sloppy drunk. Come to think of it, being drunk isn't a favorable look on *any* of us. Unless you can hold your

KNOW YOUR NUMBER

Pace yourself within it. For every drink you consume, match it with a pint or more of water. Partying is a race where first place always loses. This is not a sprint.

EAT SOMETHING

Noshing while drinking slows alcohol absorption into the bloodstream. And it'll help prevent the craving for an unhealthy fourth meal.

SAY, "CHEESE"

How are you supposed to snap a selfie with your bestie if you're double-fisting drinks all night?

KNOW YOUR SQUAD GOALS

If your people are dragging you down, audit your circle. It may sting because you can't imagine a social life without them, but you might have to sync up with better peers who don't pressure you. True friends won't care how much you don't drink.

STAY SINGLE

Asking the bartender to give you more alcohol than a drink's recommended serving size can result in double trouble.

BE SAFE

Whether they're unwarrantedly clingy or a straight-up creeper, don't put yourself in a compromising position. This goes for everyone. Use the buddy system. Pro tip: A napkin over your drink isn't impenetrable.

HIT PAUSE

Time flies when you're having fun, so take a break once in a while to capture mental snapshots of the amazing night you're having. Being mindful of our experiences also allows us to appreciate the quality and craftsmanship of what we're consuming.

PREDICT THE FUTURE

Know when to say, "When." There are almost always indications that foreshadow that the night is about to go off script.

own hair back, it's not fair to put it on your friends to babysit you time after time.

Identifying when you need to slow down or stop drinking to save the rest of your night is an investment in tomorrow. Don't make a different decision just because tomorrow is Saturday or Sunday or a day without class or work. Regardless of your commitments, no one ever says, "You know what would've made last night so much better? More shots!" A simple, "No, thanks, I'm good" is all you need to say. Knowing yourself, what you're drinking, and in what context can set you up to thrive in a lifestyle that flourishes.

> **"**
> Identifying when you need to slow down or stop drinking to save the rest of your night is an investment in tomorrow.

PART 3

BETTER
DRINKING
CULTURE

We believe in a better drinking culture. See what we did there? BDC's philosophy is rooted in *better* health, *better* relationships, and *better* communities. We're redefining *drinking*—making moderation aspirational—achievable by mindful intention in being aware of yourself, what you're consuming, and the environment around you. When blended together (stirred, not shaken), we have the opportunity to reinvigorate our *culture* with a restored promise for a healthier future.

Culture is where the rubber meets the road. Truthfully, a long road at that. A positive shift in our culture will require our joint efforts. And, if we truly desire a better drinking culture, we've got to be prepared to live it, respect it, and protect it.

7 LIVE IT

Living a BDC lifestyle does not mean you have to achieve a perfect score, but if you want to put any points on the board you have to at least participate. We will drop the ball or strike out sometimes. But, it's our decision whether we swing with intent or get sloppy at our next at bat. As leaders

> **"**
> We should be mindful of modeling a higher standard of behavior and upholding a better set of expectations.

of our peers and pioneers of change, we should be mindful of modeling a higher standard of behavior and upholding a better set of expectations.

ETIQUETTE

Let's get back to the basics. "Please." "Thank you." "You're welcome." You may think this is too elementary, but if you're ever on the other side of the bar serving instead of drinking, it will be disappointing how many people left their manners at home. Treat your friends, your peers, and the service staff with respect and common decency. This stuff matters, and makes a difference.

Etiquette is not limited to only those times when we've got a drink in our hand. It's applicable to any social situation when we're anywhere doing anything. So yeah, pretty much all the time. Think house parties, work functions, a first date, the ninety-ninth date, family gatherings, tailgating, and yes—even spring break. There are essentially two core rules to follow, on which all others are based. If you nail them, you're golden.

Rule #1: Be self-aware.
Rule #2: Be considerate of others.

For the uninitiated as well as those who could use a refresher, here are some real life, honest do-and-don't recommendations for how to etiquette better when you're out drinking.

DO

→ Have your ID ready at the door and when you order (and don't cop an attitude when asked for it or if you can't produce it). You know how it goes: Don't leave home without your ID, money, and phone.

→ Act like you're glad to be there. Going out should be a celebration, something to look forward to. Positive energy is a magnet that people want to gravitate toward.

→ Know what you want to order, or in the very least be able to give your bartender or server some direction about what you're in the mood for, what you like, and/or what you don't. If the place is slammed, they don't have time to play 20 Questions.

→ Order your drink(s) in succinct fashion. The more randomly you rattle off a confusing round of drinks, the longer it's going to take to get delivered.

→ Say, "Please" and "Thank you" when you order. Even if the bartender or server dismisses it with an unappreciative, monotone, "Yep," be the customer someone wants to wait on.

→ Tip. Rule of thumb: $1 per drink or 20% of your tab. Pro tip: If you plan to be at the same spot for longer than one-and-done, and can spare an extra buck or two, tip generously on your first drink or round. If the service warrants it, of course. You might be surprised what happens.

→ Be ready to pay when you're ready to cash out. Some establishments may require you to "pay as you go," while others may swipe your credit card (and/or hang onto it behind the bar) to start a tab. Make friendly, direct eye contact or have cash or a card patiently laid out in front of you to signal you're ready for your tab.

→ Say, "Behind!" when you're close to anyone on staff who's got their hands full. It's industry speak for, "Hey, I'm behind you, and I don't want you to drop what you're carrying." It could be your drink.

→ Leave when you're done eating or drinking, especially if the place is packed and you're occupying prime real estate. Otherwise, you're burning their table. Remember the last time you had to wait for a table longer than you were quoted?

→ Politely refuse a drink if you're not feelin' it, and don't feel like you have to justify it. Sometimes we're just not in the mood.

→ Treat everyone in the place equally regardless of gender, skin color, or any other factor of diversity. Be careful about making assumptions and judging others.

→ Leave a positive review online. Share good.

DON'T

→ Think you're the only customer in the place. Remember Rule #1?

→ Negotiate prices. Just please.

→ Pay for your drinks with sweaty dollar bills you just fished out of your bra. No you didn't...

→ Wave your money or credit card at the bartender or server, and then complain why it's taking so long to get a drink. Now, they're making you wait.

→ Ask for a free shot on your birthday. By the way, happy birthday!

→ Puff out your chest and whine, "Do you know how much money I've spent in here tonight?!" If you have to ask, the staff isn't impressed.

→ Break anything or make a mess at your table. You're an adult. There's a garbage can over there.

→ Destroy or vandalize the bathroom. Get it in the toilet or urinal. And leave the Sharpie at home.

→ Bother the DJ or band. Let them do their job. If you want to request a song, be nice about it. If they don't play it, be nice about it. And, never touch their equipment.

→ Grill someone about why they aren't drinking. It's their choice, and none of your business. Respect it. End of story.

→ Film your friends while they're drunk. Help them instead of embarrass them. No one wants to go viral like that.

→ Start a fight. It's not worth it. Be the bigger person. Walk away.

→ Be a jerk if you're ever refused service because you're too intoxicated. Laws against selling, serving, or providing alcohol to anyone visibly intoxicated are in place to protect you, the establishment, and others. Accept a water humbly.

→ Run to social media to bash a business. If you had a bad experience, especially if you were intoxicated, it very well could've been on you—not them. Contrary to popular belief, the customer is not always right.

Etiquette should not be reserved just for fancy dinner parties and black tie affairs attended exclusively by wealthy sirs and madams. Believe it or not, treating others the way you would like them to do unto you on a daily basis costs zero dollars. It's easy and abundantly available at all times. The Golden Rule is one of the most basic tenets of just being a good human, and disproves the saying that nice guys or girls finish last. You can still be cool and attractive AND nice and considerate at the same time. Crazy, right?!

8 RESPECT IT

Getting drunk requires very little skill, if any. Realize that allowing alcohol to be the central activity in which all other decisions are made puts its value above your own well-being. Drinking mindfully is a show of strength, bravery, and courage. So is asking for and accepting help when the struggle is real. It tells others that you are worth more than another drink that you may not need. For those of us who

> **"**
> Drinking mindfully is a show of strength, bravery, and courage.

respect alcohol and our own relationship with it, it's a gift to be able to share this practical wisdom with those around us. You're not selling a used car that you know is a lemon. You're telling people that the quality of the brakes on a car matter just as much as how fast it can go.

WE PLEDGE TO LOVE, SUPPORT, AND RESPECT ALL PEOPLE REGARDLESS OF THEIR RELATIONSHIP WITH ALCOHOL

Choosing not to drink for any reason, for any length of time, can sometimes be—yet shouldn't—an awkward decision to make or defend. What can be even more uncomfortable is having to address an issue when a friend might be struggling in their relationship with alcohol.

For the social drinker who occasionally stumbles, or the habitual drinker who can never seem to get up once they're down, experiencing shame is common, overwhelming, and suffocating. Just because we have a failure does not mean we are one. The rates of suicide and attempted suicide in every scenario among those who abuse alcohol are considerably higher than those of the general population.[51] Generally, we're aware enough to recognize our missteps, but confronting them can be much more of a delicate issue, and requires sensitivity. People need our love and support more than finger-pointing and ridicule. Rather than throw stones, shower others with hugs. Press in, and show you care.

Worst case scenario, if the situation goes sideways and someone is in danger—physical, mental, or otherwise—get help. Their safety should be your first priority. Someone else's suffering is not an exploitable opportunity. We need to step up and be accountable, *ESPECIALLY* if we've contributed to their intoxication.

It's not going to be fun, but you don't get to help make a mess then walk away without helping to clean it up. In those instances when we might've had too many and are unable to make coherent decisions for ourselves, our friends should step in rather than split when the going gets tough. No one deserves to be surrounded by a chalk outline of empty beer cans after they've passed out. We can't allow this to happen, or make fun of it when it does. Be each other's accountabilibuddy. Have each other's back. We've got yours. You will be respected more for telling better stories than being an accomplice to the regrettable ones.

PRINCIPLES OF RESPECTING A BETTER DRINKING CULTURE

→ Be kind. Your compassion could change someone's life.

→ Live with integrity. Do the right thing because it's the right thing to do.

→ Be honest. You'll never have to remember anything.

→ Show empathy. Be the Grinch *after* his heart grew three sizes that day.

→ Be grateful for what you have. Less is more. Unless we're talking about tacos.

→ Share what you have. Bring enough for the rest of the class.

→ Stop complaining. Unless you have a solution.

→ Don't judge. Have you walked in their shoes?

→ Laugh *with* others, not *at* them.

→ Don't be a bully. Karma's a thing.

→ Refuse to be offended. Sticks and stones...

→ Be quick to forgive. We all make mistakes.

The principles on which BDC exist rise above any differences we may have. They're rooted in compassion for the wellness and betterment of others. We can serve our friends by loving them in the ways we would want to be loved. When we walk it out for ourselves, which simultaneously models it for those around us, we are poised in an unshakable stance to defend it.

9 PROTECT IT

BDC, the *movement*, started organically by a group of friends who simply cared enough about each other to want better for themselves and others. A better drinking way of life, a *culture*, however, starts and continues with you—a tribe of motivated people all seeking something better, leveraged to advance this shared idea.

"WE MUST PROTECT THIS HOUSE!"

We all have a stake in this, which shouldn't be taken for granted. What we're building together we cannot let anyone dismantle. We will be tested, laughed at, and ignored. The haters will always attempt to crash the party and try to ruin a good time. The trolls hiding behind their keyboard will always look for a loophole to hijack the positive vibes. Don't take the bait of their immaturity or lack of compassion. They're likely struggling the hardest. And they need us the most. Choose love.

Whether we care to acknowledge it or not, so much of what we think, say, and do can be attributed to the power (i.e., pressure) of social influence. If we're being fair, this book can easily fall into that category. An argument probably will be made that BDC is trying to convince you of doing something so heinous as drinking better for yourself. Heaven forbid.

We make no bones about our mission because there isn't a victim or loser in the equation. We will not hide, shy away from, or apologize for wanting better for ourselves and others. Nor will we sacrifice our integrity so someone can stick a politically correct label on us. We're having a conversation that makes some folks uncomfortable because BDC doesn't fit neatly into their safe, default boxes. While BDC addresses the problem before it becomes one (or worse), those same people will continue to wonder why their band-aid on a wound gushing blood doesn't stop the bleeding. Nothing changes if nothing changes. This is *your choice.*

> **"**
> Let's help by not subscribing to the glamorization of binge drinking on social media.

Let's help by not subscribing to the glamorization of binge drinking on social media and anywhere else where no F's are given. When we engage by laughing at the pitiful scenarios

> **"**
> Our culture is thirsty for leaders to carve a better path for the next generation.

characteristic of getting wasted—when we like it, heart it, follow it, or share it—it's only a reflection on us, and we're better than that. Exhibiting restraint is a show of maturity and leadership. In a virtual, social world where

> **"**
> Shifting ourselves toward a better drinking culture will happen because of you.

funny trumps everything, stop for a moment to consider whether they're laughing with you or at you. Just because it happened, doesn't mean it's intended for the world to make fun of. The curb appeal of jumping on the bandwagon because it's popular

in the moment will quickly fade if you end up on the business end of a night out gone wrong.

Together, we become greater than the sum of our parts. We can encourage our peers to be proud of having a healthier relationship with alcohol, where binge drinking isn't socially accepted or an applauded stunt. Our culture is thirsty for leaders to carve a better path for the next generation ... the one after that ... and the one after that. You have a voice that deserves to be heard, and we have a platform on which you can stand with confidence. You are right to feel empowered, to inspire others, and to impact monumental social change in a tangible way our world has never felt.

Shifting ourselves toward a better drinking culture will happen because of you. Your decision to be courageous in doing the right thing—the *better* thing—for yourself, your loved ones, and your inner circle carries weight and momentum into the next generation. Your choice to drink better is meaningful and contributes to a bigger purpose that our culture needs and our friends deserve. You get to be the author of your own story. You have every bit of authority to write it in such a way that either changes the dynamic of our culture or succumbs to it.

Your move.

SOURCES

CHAPTER 1

1. European College of Neuropsychopharmacology. "Can You Avoid Hangovers After Heavy Drinking?" Europe: European College of Neuropsychopharmacology, 29 August 2015. ecnp.eu/~/media/Files/ecnp/About%20ECNP/Press/AMS2015/Verster%20pr%20FINAL.pdf.

2. "Alcohol and Ibuprofen: Can You Mix Ibuprofen and Alcohol?" The Recovery Village, therecoveryvillage.com/alcohol-abuse/alcohol-and-ibuprofen/#gref.

3. Dresden, Danielle. "What is the Hippocampus?" *Medical News Today*. 7 December 2017, medicalnewstoday.com/articles/313295.php.

4. Ebrahim, lrshaad, et al. "Alcohol and Sleep Review: Sound Statistics and Valid Conclusions," *Alcoholism: Clinical and Experimental Research*, vol. 39, no. 5, 2015, pp. 944-946. Wiley Online Library, doi.org/10.1111/acer.12708.

5. Cuffey, Abigail. "How Alcohol Messes With Your Sleep -- And What You Can Do About It." Huffington Post. 10 July 2017, huffingtonpost.com/entry/how-alcohol-affects-sleep_us_595fbd02e4b0615b9e91273c.

6. Ebrahim, lrshaad, et al. "Alcohol and Sleep Review: Sound Statistics and Valid Conclusions," *Alcoholism: Clinical and Experimental Research*, vol. 39, no. 5, 2015, pp. 944-946. Wiley Online Library, doi.org/10.1111/acer.12708.

7. Wechsler, H., et al. "Changes in Binge Drinking and Related Problems Among American College Students Between 1993 and 1997: Results of

the Harvard School of Public Health College Alcohol Study." *Journal of American College Health*, vol. 47, no. 2, 1998, pp. 57-68. National Center for Biotechnology Information, doi: 10.1080/07448489809595621, ncbi.nlm. nih.gov/pubmed/9782661.

8. Wyatt, Gary. "Skipping Class: An Analysis of Absenteeism Among First-Year College Students." *Teaching Sociology*, vol. 20, no. 3, 17 July 1992, pp. 201-07. ResearchGate, doi: 10.2307/1319061, researchgate.net/publication/272588439_Skipping_Class_An_Analysis_of_Absenteeism_among_First-Year_College_Students.

9. Stoddard, Tim. "College Kids and Alcohol Abuse - Just How Serious Is It?" Sober Nation. 23 December 2014. sobernation.com/college-kids-and-alcohol-abuse/.

10. Porter, S.R., & Pryor, J. "The Effects of Heavy Episodic Alcohol Use on Student Engagement, Academic Performance, and Time Use." *Journal of College Student Development*, vol. 48, no. 4, 2007, pp. 455-467. *PsycNET*, dx.doi.org/10.1353/csd.2007.0042.

11. Wechsler, H., et al. "Changes in Binge Drinking and Related Problems Among American College Students Between 1993 and 1997: Results of the Harvard School of Public Health College Alcohol Study." *Journal of American College Health*, vol. 47, no. 2, 1998, pp. 57-68. National Center for Biotechnology Information, doi: 10.1080/07448489809595621, ncbi.nlm. nih.gov/pubmed/9782661.

12. Porter, S.R., & Pryor, J. "The Effects of Heavy Episodic Alcohol Use on Student Engagement, Academic Performance, and Time Use." *Journal of College Student Development*, vol. 48, no. 4, 2007, pp. 455-467.

13. Thombs, D.L., et al. "Undergraduate Drinking and Academic Performance: A Prospective Investigation with Objective Measures." *Journal of Studies on Alcohol and Drugs*. vol. 70, no. 5, 2009, pp. 776-785.

14. Presley, C.A., et al. "Alcohol and Drugs on American College Campuses: Use, Consequences, and Perceptions of the Campus Environment." vol 1:

1989-1991, 1993. ERIC, eric.ed.gov/?id=ED358766.

15. Wolaver, A. "Effect of Heavy Drinking in College on Student Effort, Grade Point Average, and Major Choice." *Contemporary Economic Policy*, vol. 20, no. 4, 2002, pp. 415-428. Wiley Online Library, doi.org/10.1093/cep/20.4.415.

16. Firth, Gina and Manzo, Luis. "For the Athlete: Alcohol and Athletic Performance." University of Notre Dame, 2004.

17. "Alcohol Facts and Statistics." *National Institute on Alcohol Abuse and Alcoholism*, niaaa.nih.gov/alcohol-health/overview-alcohol-consumption/alcohol-facts-and-statistics.

18. "Addiction Medicine: Closing the Gap Between Science and Practice." Casa Columbia, 2012, centeronaddiction.org/addiction/addiction-risk-factors.

19. Russell, M. "Prevalence of Alcoholism Among Children of Alcoholics." *Children of Alcoholics: Critical Perspectives*. New York: Guilford, 1990, pp. 9-38, pubs.niaaa.nih.gov/publications/AA67/AA67.htm.

20. Hatfield, Rudy. "Warning Signs of Addiction." *Project Know*, projectknow.com/research/addiction-warning-signs/.

21. "Alcohol Addiction." *Project Know*, projectknow.com/research/alcohol-addiction/.

22. "Understanding the Difference Between Alcohol Use and Alcoholism." The Recovery Village, 16 May 2017, therecoveryvillage.com/recovery-blog/alcoholism-alcohol-use-disorder-whats-difference/.

23. Blanco, C., et al. "Mental Health of College Students and Their Non-College-Attending Peers: Results from the National Epidemiologic Study on Alcohol and Related Conditions. *Archives of General Psychiatry*. vol. 65, no. 12, 2008, pp. 1429-1437, PMID: 19047530, ncbi.nlm.nih.gov/pmc/articles/PMC2734947/.

24. "Addiction Medicine: Closing the Gap between Science and Practice." *Center on Addiction*, June 2012, centeronaddiction.org/addiction-research/reports/addiction-medicine-closing-gap-between-science-and-practice.

25. "Teen Substance Use." *Center on Addiction*, centeronaddiction.org/addiction-prevention/teenage-addiction.

26. *Center for Behavioral Health Statistics and Quality.* "2015 National Survey on Drug Use and Health: Detailed Tables." Substance Abuse and Mental Health Services Administration, Rockville, MD, 2016.

27. "Underage Drinking." *National Institute on Alcohol and Alcoholism*, pubs.niaaa.nih.gov/publications/UnderageDrinking/UnderageFact.htm.

28. "Underage Drinking." *National Institute on Alcohol and Alcoholism*, pubs.niaaa.nih.gov/publications/UnderageDrinking/UnderageFact.htm.

CHAPTER 2

29. "Alcohol and Aggression." Drinkaware, drinkaware.co.uk/alcohol-facts/health-effects-of-alcohol/mental-health/alcohol-and-aggression/.

30. "Alcohol, Drugs and Crime." National Council on Alcoholism and Drug Dependence, Inc., ncadd.org/about-addiction/alcohol-drugs-and-crime.

31. "Alcohol, Drugs and Crime." National Council on Alcoholism and Drug Dependence, Inc., ncadd.org/about-addiction/alcohol-drugs-and-crime.

32. Hingson R., et al. "Magnitude of Alcohol-Related Mortality and Morbidity Among U.S. College Students Ages 18–24: Changes from 1998 to 2001." *Annual Review of Public Health*, vol. 26, 2005, pp. 259-279. National Center for Biotechnology Information, annualreviews.org/doi/10.1146/annurev.publhealth.26.021304.144652.

33. Wechsler, H., et al. "Changes in Binge Drinking and Related Problems

Among American College Students Between 1993 and 1997: Results of the Harvard School of Public Health College Alcohol Study." *Journal of American College Health*, vol. 47, no. 2, 1998, pp. 57-68. National Center for Biotechnology Information, annualreviews.org/doi/10.1146/annurev. publhealth.26.021304.144652.

34. Join Together Online, intheknowzone.com/substance-abuse-topics/ binge-drinking/statistics.html.

35. "Alcohol Effects On Performance Monitoring and Adjustment: Affect Modulation and Impairment of Evaluative Cognitive Control." *Journal of Abnormal Psychology*, vol. 121, no. 1, February 2012, pp. 173-186. National Center for Biotechnology Information, doi: 10.1037/a0023664.

CHAPTER 3

36. Sacks, J.J., et al. "2010 National and State Costs of Excessive Alcohol Consumption." *American Journal of Preventive Medicine*, vol. 49, no. 5, 2015, pp.73-79. doi.org/10.1016/j.amepre.2015.05.03.

37. "Alcohol Facts and Statistics." *National Institute on Alcohol Abuse and Alcoholism*, niaaa.nih.gov/alcohol-health/overview-alcohol-consumption/ alcohol-facts-and-statistics.

38. "Alcohol Facts and Statistics." *National Institute on Alcohol Abuse and Alcoholism*, niaaa.nih.gov/alcohol-health/overview-alcohol-consumption/ alcohol-facts-and-statistics.

39. "Alcohol and Sexual Assault." *National Institute on Alcohol Abuse and Alcoholism*, pubs.niaaa.nih.gov/publications/arh25-1/43-51.htm.

40. "Alcohol, Drugs and Crime." *National Council on Alcoholism and Drug Dependence, Inc.*, ncadd.org/about-addiction/alcohol-drugs-and-crime.

41. "Alcohol, Drugs and Crime." *National Council on Alcoholism and Drug Dependence, Inc.*, ncadd.org/about-addiction/alcohol-drugs-and-crime.

42. "Traffic Safety Facts 2016 Data: Alcohol-Impaired Driving." *National Highway Traffic Safety Administration: U.S. Department of Transportation*, 2017, https://crashstats.nhtsa.dot.gov/Api/Public/ViewPublication/812450.

43. "Fact Sheets - Alcohol Use and Your Health." *Centers for Disease Control and Prevention*, cdc.gov/alcohol/fact-sheets/alcohol-use.pdf.

CHAPTER 4

44. Boden, Joseph and David Fergusson. "Alcohol and Depression." *Addiction*, vol. 106, no. 5, March 2011, pp. 906-914. Research Gate, doi: 10.1111/j.1360-0443.2010.03351.x, researchgate.net/publication/50303291_Alcohol_and_depression.

45. "Alcohol and Depression." *WebMD*, webmd.com/depression/guide/alcohol-and-depresssion#1-2.

CHAPTER 5

46. U.S. Department of Health and Human Services. *Dietary Guidelines for Americans: 2015-2020, Appendix 9*, health.gov/dietaryguidelines/2015/guidelines/appendix-9/.

47. Frezza, M. ; Di Padova, C.; Pozzato, G.; et al. "High Blood Alcohol Levels In Women: The Role of Decreased Gastric Alcohol Dehydrogenase Activity and First-Pass Metabolism." *New England Journal of Medicine*, vol. 322, no. 2, 1990, pubs.niaaa.nih.gov/publications/aa46.htm.

48. "Blood Alcohol Concentration (BAC)." In the Know Zone, intheknowzone.com/substance-abuse-topics/alcohol/bac.html.

49. "Alcohol Poisoning Deaths." *Centers for Disease Control and Prevention*, cdc.gov/vitalsigns/alcohol-poisoning-deaths/index.html.

50. "Alcohol Poisoning Deaths." *Centers for Disease Control and Prevention*,

cdc.gov/vitalsigns/alcohol-poisoning-deaths/index.html.

CHAPTER 8

51. "The Association Between Alcohol Misuse and Suicidal Behaviour." *Alcohol and Alcoholism*, vol. 41, no. 5, 1 September 2006, pp. 473-478, doi. org/10.1093/alcalc/agl060.

BUILDING A BETTER DRINKING CULTURE

MORNINGS ARE BETTER WITHOUT HANGOVERS. LIFE IS BETTER WITHOUT REGRETS. LIFE IS TOO SHORT TO FORGET WHAT HAPPENED LAST NIGHT. WE EMBRACE QUALITY OVER QUANTITY. WE ENCOURAGE CHOICES THAT REDUCE OUR RISK FOR ADDICTION. WE PLEDGE TO LOVE, SUPPORT, AND RESPECT ALL PEOPLE REGARDLESS OF THEIR RELATIONSHIP WITH ALCOHOL.

ALCOHOL SHOULD

- NEVER TURN US INTO SOMEONE WE'RE NOT
- NEVER HURT RELATIONSHIPS
- NEVER PUT OURSELVES OR OTHERS IN HARM'S WAY
- BE A CHOICE—NOT AN EXPECTATION
- BE A CRAFT THAT'S ENJOYED—NOT A TOOL FOR DEALING WITH LIFE

BETTER DRINKING CULTURE

DRINK BETTER. LIVE HEALTHIER.
#BECAUSEHANGOVERSSUCK

BETTERDRINKINGCULTURE.ORG